Kyphosis Made Clear

How To Take Charge Of Your Spinal Health And Improve

Your Posture Permanently

DR. BRODY ATTICUS

Table of Contents

Introductory

Our spine is one of the most remarkable structures in the human body — a flexible yet strong column of bones, discs, ligaments, and muscles that supports our weight, allows movement, and protects the delicate spinal cord. From the side, a healthy spine has natural curves: a slight inward curve at the neck (cervical lordosis), an outward curve at the upper back (thoracic kyphosis), and another inward curve in the lower back (lumbar lordosis). These gentle curves act as shock absorbers, balancing the body and helping us move with ease.

Kyphosis is a term used to describe an exaggerated outward curvature of the thoracic spine, leading to a rounded or hunched appearance of the upper back. While some curvature is normal — typically between 20° and 50° — kyphosis refers to cases where the curvature exceeds the healthy range, altering posture and, in more severe situations, impacting movement, breathing, and quality of life.

Kyphosis is not a single condition but a descriptive term that can have many causes, patterns, and severities. It may develop gradually over years due to **age-related spinal changes**, or appear suddenly after **trauma, fractures, or underlying medical disorders**. Some people are born with structural differences in their vertebrae, leading to **congenital kyphosis**, while others develop **postural kyphosis** in adolescence, often linked to prolonged poor posture, muscle imbalances, or habits in a technology-driven world.

Although kyphosis is sometimes dismissed as a "posture problem" or a harmless part of aging, its impact can be far-reaching. Beyond the visible changes in body shape, kyphosis can cause **back pain, muscle fatigue, stiffness, reduced flexibility, and even respiratory or neurological complications** in advanced cases. Psychologically, it may influence self-image, confidence, and social comfort, especially in teenagers and young adults.

Understanding kyphosis requires looking beyond the curve itself. It is about **how the vertebrae are shaped**, **how the muscles support the spine**, and **how lifestyle, health conditions, and genetics interact** to shape spinal health over time. Early recognition and proactive management are essential — not only because certain types of kyphosis can worsen if untreated, but because the spine is deeply connected to our overall well-being.

Thankfully, kyphosis is not always a fixed or permanent condition. In many cases, targeted exercises, postural training, bracing, and lifestyle changes can improve alignment and slow progression. Even in more severe or structural cases, modern treatments — including surgical options when necessary — can restore function and reduce discomfort.

The key is **awareness, timely intervention, and a holistic approach** that considers both the physical and emotional effects of the condition.

This book aims to **demystify kyphosis**, separating myth from fact, and providing clear, evidence-based guidance for prevention, diagnosis, and treatment. You will learn:

- How to recognize early signs and symptoms of kyphosis.
- The different types — from postural to structural — and how they develop.
- The role of muscles, ligaments, bones, and lifestyle habits in spinal curvature.
- When medical evaluation is necessary and what diagnostic tests involve.
- Practical, safe exercises and ergonomic strategies to support spinal health.
- Emotional coping strategies for dealing with visible posture changes.

Whether you are a patient, caregiver, healthcare provider, or simply someone concerned about spinal health, understanding kyphosis is the first step toward taking control.

CHAPTER ONE: UNDERSTANDING YOUR SPINE

The Anatomy Of The Spine

To understand kyphosis and how it affects posture and spinal health, it is essential first to grasp the structure, function, and mechanics of the spine. The spine, also known as the vertebral column or backbone, is a complex, dynamic structure that supports the body, enables movement, and protects the spinal cord — the main communication highway between the brain and the rest of the body.

1.1 Overview of the Spine: The human spine consists of **33 vertebrae** stacked one atop another, separated by **intervertebral discs**, and connected by **ligaments** and **muscles**. It is divided into five distinct regions:

Cervical Spine (Neck):

- Composed of 7 vertebrae (C1–C7).
- Supports the head and allows for a wide range of motion — flexion, extension, rotation, and lateral bending.
- The first two vertebrae, the **atlas (C1)** and **axis (C2)**, are uniquely shaped to enable head rotation.

Thoracic Spine (Upper and Mid-Back):

- Made up of 12 vertebrae (T1–T12).
- Forms the natural outward curve called **kyphosis** in healthy posture (20°–50°).
- Each vertebra articulates with the ribs, providing structural support and protecting vital organs in the chest.
- Less flexible than the cervical and lumbar regions, but essential for stability.

Lumbar Spine (Lower Back):

- Contains 5 vertebrae (L1–L5).
- Bears the weight of the upper body and allows significant flexibility in bending and twisting.
- Naturally curves inward (**lordosis**) to distribute forces efficiently.

Sacrum:

- A triangular-shaped bone formed by the fusion of 5 vertebrae (S1–S5).
- Connects the spine to the pelvis, stabilizing the body during standing and walking.

Coccyx (Tailbone):

- Comprised of 3–5 fused vertebrae.
- Serves as an attachment point for ligaments and muscles of the pelvic floor.

1.2 Intervertebral Discs: Between most vertebrae lie **intervertebral discs**, which act as cushions, absorbing shock and allowing flexibility. Each disc has two main parts:

- **Nucleus pulposus:** The gel-like center that provides elasticity.
- **Annulus fibrosus:** The tough outer layer that holds the nucleus in place and resists excessive movement.

Healthy discs are crucial for proper spinal alignment. Degeneration or damage to these discs can contribute to abnormal spinal curvatures, including kyphosis.

1.3 Ligaments and Muscles: The spine is reinforced by **ligaments**, which connect bones and stabilize the vertebral column, and **muscles**, which control movement and posture. Key muscles include:

- **Erector spinae:** Runs along the spine, maintaining upright posture.
- **Multifidus:** Stabilizes individual vertebrae.

- **Abdominal muscles:** Support the spine from the front, balancing the forces from the back muscles.

Imbalances or weakness in these muscles can contribute to postural kyphosis and spinal discomfort.

1.4 Spinal Curves and Their Function: A healthy spine has natural curves that form an **S-shape** when viewed from the side:

- **Cervical lordosis**: inward curve of the neck.
- **Thoracic kyphosis**: outward curve of the upper back.
- **Lumbar lordosis**: inward curve of the lower back.

These curves act as shock absorbers, distribute mechanical stress, and help maintain balance. When the thoracic curve becomes exaggerated, it results in **kyphosis**, affecting posture, mobility, and overall spinal health.

1.5 The Spinal Cord and Nerves: The spinal cord runs through the **vertebral canal**, protected by the vertebrae. Nerves branch out from the spinal cord through openings called **intervertebral foramina**, connecting the brain to every part of the body. Damage, compression, or deformity in the spine — such as that caused by severe kyphosis — can interfere with nerve function, leading to pain, weakness, or sensory changes.

The spine is a delicate balance of strength and flexibility, designed to support movement, protect the nervous system, and maintain posture. Understanding its anatomy — vertebrae, discs, ligaments, muscles, curves, and nerves — is the foundation for recognizing, preventing, and managing spinal conditions like kyphosis. Knowledge of these structures allows for better assessment of posture, early identification of spinal abnormalities, and targeted interventions to maintain spinal health for life.

Defining Kyphosis: Normal Vs. Excessive Curvature

Kyphosis refers to the outward curvature of the thoracic (upper and mid-back) portion of the spine. While a slight outward curve is a normal and essential part of healthy spinal anatomy, excessive curvature can lead to postural changes, discomfort, and functional limitations.

Normal Thoracic Curvature:

In a healthy spine, the thoracic region naturally curves outward between **20° and 50°**. This normal kyphotic curve helps:

- Absorb shock during movement
- Maintain proper balance and alignment
- Protect the spinal cord and internal organs

This mild curve is considered normal and typically does not cause pain or interfere with mobility.

Excessive Kyphosis:

Excessive kyphosis occurs when the thoracic curve exceeds the normal range, often resulting in a **rounded or hunched upper back**. Depending on severity, it may cause:

- Visible postural changes, such as a hump or forward-slumping shoulders
- Muscle fatigue and stiffness
- Pain in the back, neck, or shoulders
- Reduced flexibility and mobility

In severe cases, breathing or spinal nerve complications

Types of Kyphosis:

Excessive kyphosis can develop for various reasons:

- **Postural kyphosis:** Often caused by poor posture, muscle weakness, or prolonged slouching, common in adolescents.
- **Structural kyphosis:** Results from changes in vertebrae, such as fractures, congenital abnormalities, or degenerative diseases.

- **Scheuermann's kyphosis:** A developmental condition during adolescence, where vertebrae grow unevenly, creating a more pronounced curve.

Understanding the difference between normal and excessive kyphotic curvature is essential for early recognition and intervention. While mild curvature is natural and healthy, persistent or worsening excessive curvature should be evaluated by a healthcare professional to prevent long-term complications.

Types Of Kyphosis: Postural, Scheuermann's, Congenital, And Osteoporotic

Kyphosis is not a single condition but a term describing an excessive outward curvature of the thoracic spine. Understanding the different types is crucial for identifying causes, determining severity, and selecting appropriate management strategies. The most common forms of kyphosis include **postural, Scheuermann's, congenital, and osteoporotic**.

1. Postural Kyphosis: Postural kyphosis is the most common form, often associated with poor posture, prolonged slouching, or muscle weakness. It typically develops during adolescence and is more prevalent in individuals who spend long periods sitting or using electronic devices.

Key characteristics:

- The curvature is flexible and can often be corrected by consciously straightening the back.
- Usually painless, though prolonged slouching may lead to muscle fatigue.
- Rarely causes neurological or spinal complications.

Management:

- Postural training and strengthening exercises for the back and core muscles.
- Ergonomic adjustments to daily activities and school or work environments.
- In most cases, no surgery is needed.

2. Scheuermann's Kyphosis: Scheuermann's kyphosis is a structural form of kyphosis that develops during adolescence due to abnormal vertebral growth. In this condition, the vertebrae become wedge-shaped, causing a more rigid and pronounced spinal curve.

Key characteristics:

- Usually presents in teenagers, often worsening during growth spurts.
- The curve is more rigid than postural kyphosis and does not fully correct with posture changes.
- May cause back pain, stiffness, and fatigue with activity.

Management:

- Physical therapy focusing on flexibility and strength.
- Bracing in moderate cases to prevent progression.
- Surgery in severe cases to correct curvature and relieve symptoms.

3. Congenital Kyphosis: Congenital kyphosis results from spinal malformations present at birth, caused by abnormal vertebral development in the womb. This form of kyphosis is structural and usually becomes more apparent as the child grows.

Key characteristics:

- Can vary from mild to severe, depending on the extent of vertebral malformation.
- May be associated with other spinal or systemic abnormalities.
- The curve is rigid and often progressive if untreated.

Management:

- Early monitoring and imaging to assess progression.
- Surgical intervention may be necessary to prevent severe deformity or neurological complications.
- Physical therapy may support overall spinal function.

4. Osteoporotic Kyphosis: Osteoporotic kyphosis occurs in adults, most commonly in older women, due to **vertebral compression fractures** caused by osteoporosis. Weakening of the vertebrae allows them to collapse, increasing the thoracic curve.

Key characteristics:

- Gradual onset, often noticed as a stooped posture or "dowager's hump."
- May cause chronic back pain, decreased mobility, and reduced height.
- In severe cases, can impact lung function and quality of life.

Management:

- Osteoporosis treatment, including medications to strengthen bones.
- Physical therapy to maintain mobility and strengthen supporting muscles.
- Bracing in some cases to stabilize the spine.

- Surgery may be necessary in severe fractures or progressive deformity.

Kyphosis can result from a variety of causes, from poor posture to congenital or degenerative spinal changes. Recognizing the type of kyphosis is essential for developing an effective treatment plan, improving posture, preventing progression, and maintaining overall spinal health. While some forms are flexible and correctable with lifestyle changes, others require medical or surgical intervention to prevent complications.

How Kyphosis Develops Over Time

Kyphosis is not typically a sudden condition. Instead, it often develops gradually over months or years, influenced by factors such as age, posture, spinal health, and underlying medical conditions. Understanding the progression of kyphosis is essential for early recognition, timely intervention, and effective management.

1. Early Stage: Subtle Changes: In the early stages, kyphosis may be barely noticeable. The outward curvature of the thoracic spine is mild, and many individuals experience no pain or functional limitations. Common early signs include:

- Slight rounding of the upper back

- Mild fatigue or discomfort after prolonged sitting or standing
- Leaning forward when walking or standing for long periods

At this stage, the curve is often flexible, particularly in cases of postural kyphosis. Awareness, posture correction, and targeted exercises can prevent further progression.

2. Progressive Stage: Noticeable Curvature: As kyphosis develops further, the curvature becomes more pronounced and harder to correct voluntarily. This stage can occur due to:

- Persistent poor posture and muscle weakness
- Structural changes in the vertebrae (Scheuermann's or congenital kyphosis)
- Vertebral compression from osteoporosis in older adults
- Symptoms may begin to appear, including:
- Visible rounding or "hunchback" appearance
- Back, neck, or shoulder discomfort
- Decreased flexibility and reduced ability to stand upright for long periods

Progression may be slow over several years, but in certain cases — such as rapid growth during adolescence or post-fracture collapse in osteoporosis — kyphosis can worsen more quickly.

3. Advanced Stage: Severe Curvature and Complications: In severe kyphosis, the thoracic curve exceeds normal limits significantly, which may lead to functional and health complications:

- Chronic pain and muscle fatigue due to altered spinal mechanics
- Limited mobility and difficulty performing daily activities
- Potential impact on lung function, causing shortness of breath
- Rarely, compression of the spinal cord or nerve roots, leading to neurological symptoms such as tingling, numbness, or weakness

At this stage, kyphosis may become structural, meaning the curvature cannot be fully corrected by posture changes alone. Medical evaluation and targeted interventions, including bracing or surgery in extreme cases, are often required.

4. Factors Influencing Progression: Several factors can accelerate the development of kyphosis over time:

- **Age-related degeneration:** Weakening of vertebrae and discs can increase curvature.
- **Bone health:** Osteoporosis or vertebral fractures contribute to progression.
- **Muscle strength:** Weak back and core muscles reduce spinal support.

- **Lifestyle habits:** Prolonged slouching, heavy backpacks, or sedentary behavior exacerbate postural kyphosis.
- **Genetic or congenital conditions:** Structural vertebral abnormalities can worsen as the child grows.

5. Early Recognition and Prevention: Early detection is critical to preventing severe kyphosis. Regular monitoring of posture, awareness of back discomfort, and attention to spinal health can help identify subtle changes before they progress. Interventions such as postural exercises, core strengthening, ergonomic adjustments, and treatment of underlying conditions are most effective when implemented early.

Kyphosis is a dynamic condition that develops gradually over time. While some forms remain mild and manageable, others can progress to severe curvature with physical and functional consequences. Recognizing the stages of kyphosis — from subtle postural changes to advanced spinal deformity — allows for timely intervention, improved posture, and long-term spinal health.

Signs, Symptoms, And Early Detection Of Kyphosis

Recognizing kyphosis early is crucial for effective management and prevention of complications. While some forms of kyphosis are mild and painless, others can progress over time, causing discomfort, postural changes, and functional limitations. Understanding the signs and symptoms allows individuals and healthcare providers to intervene before the curvature becomes severe.

1. Visible Signs of Kyphosis: One of the earliest indicators of kyphosis is a noticeable change in posture. Common visual signs include:

- **Rounded or hunched upper back:** The thoracic spine appears excessively curved.
- **Forward head posture:** The head may jut forward to compensate for the upper back curve.
- **Shoulder drooping or rounding:** Shoulders may slouch forward.
- **Uneven or slanted shoulders or hips:** In structural kyphosis, vertebral asymmetry may cause imbalance.
- **Loss of height over time:** Progressive curvature can result in a measurable decrease in overall height.

2. Common Symptoms: Symptoms of kyphosis vary depending on type, severity, and age. They can include:

- **Back pain or stiffness:** Often mild in postural kyphosis but more pronounced in Scheuermann's or osteoporotic kyphosis.
- **Muscle fatigue:** Prolonged standing or walking may cause fatigue in the back, neck, or shoulders.

- **Reduced flexibility:** Difficulty bending, twisting, or performing activities that require full spinal mobility.
- **Neurological symptoms (in severe cases):** Tingling, numbness, or weakness in the arms or legs due to nerve compression.
- **Respiratory issues:** In severe thoracic curvature, lung expansion may be limited, causing shortness of breath.

3. Early Detection: Early detection of kyphosis is essential to prevent progression and manage symptoms effectively. Key strategies include:

a. Self-Observation and Posture Checks:

- Stand sideways in front of a mirror and check for rounding of the upper back or forward head posture.
- Monitor for slouched shoulders, uneven shoulders or hips, or a gradual loss of height.

b. Physical Examination: Healthcare providers assess kyphosis through:

- **Visual inspection:** Evaluating the spinal curve and overall posture.
- **Flexibility tests:** Determining if the curvature is flexible (postural) or rigid (structural).
- **Palpation:** Feeling the spine and surrounding muscles for tenderness or tightness.

c. Diagnostic Imaging

- **X-rays:** Provide precise measurement of the thoracic curvature, often using the Cobb angle to quantify severity.
- **MRI or CT scans:** Used when there is concern about underlying vertebral abnormalities, spinal cord compression, or other structural issues.

4. Risk Factors for Early Detection: Certain individuals should be especially vigilant for early signs of kyphosis:

- Adolescents, particularly during growth spurts (risk for postural or Scheuermann's kyphosis)
- Older adults, especially women with osteoporosis (risk for vertebral fractures and osteoporotic kyphosis)
- Individuals with a family history of spinal deformities
- People with poor posture, sedentary lifestyle, or weak back and core muscles

5. Importance of Early Intervention: Detecting kyphosis early can prevent further curvature, reduce discomfort, and maintain functional mobility. Early interventions may include:

- Postural correction and ergonomic adjustments
- Targeted strengthening and stretching exercises

- Monitoring and treatment of underlying conditions (e.g., osteoporosis or vertebral anomalies)
- Bracing in moderate structural cases

Kyphosis often develops gradually, making early recognition critical. Visual changes in posture, back discomfort, muscle fatigue, and reduced flexibility are key warning signs. By observing these indicators and seeking timely evaluation, individuals can take proactive steps to manage kyphosis, maintain spinal health, and prevent long-term complications.

CHAPTER TWO: CAUSES AND RISK FACTORS

Posture-Related Causes Of Kyphosis

Postural habits play a significant role in the development of kyphosis, particularly in adolescents and adults who spend long periods sitting or performing repetitive activities. While a certain degree of thoracic curvature is normal, poor posture over time can exaggerate this curve, leading to **postural kyphosis**, one of the most common and preventable forms of spinal curvature.

1. Slouching and Forward Head Posture: Frequent slouching, hunching over desks, electronic devices, or smartphones can gradually increase thoracic curvature. Forward head posture often accompanies slouching, further straining the upper back muscles. Over time, this leads to:

- Weakening of postural muscles in the back
- Tightening of chest muscles
- Increased reliance on ligaments for spinal support, which can contribute to permanent curvature if uncorrected

2. Prolonged Sitting and Sedentary Lifestyle: Modern lifestyles often involve long hours sitting at computers, in classrooms, or while commuting. A sedentary lifestyle can:

- Reduce the strength and endurance of the back extensors that help maintain upright posture
- Encourage habitual rounding of the upper back
- Increase the risk of gradual, cumulative kyphotic curvature over months or years

3. Carrying Heavy Loads Improperly: Frequent lifting or carrying heavy backpacks, especially on one shoulder, can strain the spine and promote postural kyphosis. This is particularly common in school-aged children and adolescents. Improper weight distribution causes:

- Increased stress on thoracic vertebrae
- Muscle imbalances between the back and chest
- Potential development of forward rounding over time

4. Muscle Weakness and Imbalance: Posture-related kyphosis often results from **muscle imbalances**:

- **Weak back muscles**: Unable to counteract the forward pull of gravity and chest muscles
- **Tight chest muscles**: Pull the shoulders and upper back forward, exaggerating curvature
- **Weak core muscles**: Fail to provide adequate support for spinal alignment

Addressing these imbalances through strengthening and stretching is critical in preventing or correcting postural kyphosis.

5. Poor Ergonomics and Work Habits: Workstations, study areas, and daily routines can influence spinal posture. Poorly designed desks, chairs, or screens positioned too low or high encourage leaning forward and rounding of the upper back. Over time, repeated poor posture reinforces kyphotic tendencies.

6. Lifestyle Interventions: Fortunately, posture-related kyphosis is highly preventable and often reversible when detected early. Key interventions include:

- Practicing proper sitting and standing posture
- Regular exercise focusing on back, core, and chest muscles
- Adjusting workstations and electronic device positions for ergonomics
- Limiting prolonged sitting and incorporating regular movement breaks

Posture-related kyphosis develops gradually from habitual slouching, prolonged sitting, muscle weakness, and poor ergonomics. By recognizing these contributing factors and implementing corrective strategies early, individuals can maintain a healthy spinal curve, reduce discomfort, and prevent permanent deformity.

Medical And Structural Causes Of Kyphosis

While poor posture and lifestyle habits can contribute to kyphosis, many cases arise from **medical conditions or structural abnormalities** of the spine. Understanding these causes is essential for accurate diagnosis, appropriate treatment, and prevention of complications.

1. Scheuermann's Disease: Scheuermann's kyphosis is a structural form of kyphosis that typically develops during adolescence. It occurs when the **vertebrae grow unevenly**, resulting in wedge-shaped vertebrae and a rigid, pronounced curvature of the thoracic spine.

Key characteristics:

- More common in teenagers, often during growth spurts
- Curve is rigid and does not fully correct with posture changes
- May cause back pain, stiffness, and fatigue

Management:

- Physical therapy to improve flexibility and strength
- Bracing in moderate cases to prevent progression
- Surgery in severe cases

2. Congenital Kyphosis: Congenital kyphosis arises from **vertebral malformations present at birth**. Abnormal development of the vertebrae in utero can lead to a curve that becomes more pronounced as the child grows.

Key characteristics:

- May vary from mild to severe
- Often progressive if untreated
- Can be associated with other spinal or systemic abnormalities

Management:

- Early monitoring with imaging
- Surgical intervention to prevent severe deformity
- Physical therapy to maintain spinal function

3. Osteoporotic Kyphosis: Osteoporotic kyphosis is most common in older adults, particularly women, due to **vertebral compression fractures caused by weakened bones**. As the vertebrae collapse, the thoracic curve increases, resulting in the classic "dowager's hump."

Key characteristics:

- Gradual development over months or years
- Back pain and reduced mobility
- Potential impact on height, lung function, and quality of life

Management:

- Osteoporosis treatment, including medications and supplements
- Physical therapy to strengthen supporting muscles
- Bracing for spinal stabilization
- Surgery in severe cases or fractures

4. Degenerative Disc Disease and Arthritis: Age-related degeneration of spinal discs and joints can alter vertebral alignment, leading to kyphotic curvature. Conditions such as **degenerative disc disease, spondylosis, and spinal arthritis** may cause:

- Loss of disc height
- Vertebral collapse or wedging
- Stiffness and pain contributing to postural changes

Management:

- Pain management through medications or therapy
- Postural exercises and spinal stabilization
- In some cases, surgical intervention

5. Trauma and Spinal Injuries: Kyphosis can also develop following **fractures, dislocations, or severe spinal injuries**. Traumatic events may cause vertebral collapse or malalignment, leading to abnormal curvature.

Management:

- Prompt medical evaluation and imaging
- Bracing or immobilization to support healing
- Surgery in severe or unstable fractures

6. Neuromuscular and Systemic Conditions: Certain neuromuscular or systemic disorders can affect spinal development and stability, increasing the risk of kyphosis. Examples include:

- **Muscular dystrophy**: Weakens supporting muscles
- **Polio or cerebral palsy**: Alters spinal alignment
- **Connective tissue disorders**: Such as Marfan syndrome

Management focuses on addressing the underlying condition, maintaining spinal support, and monitoring curvature progression.

Medical and structural causes of kyphosis often result in **rigid, progressive curves** that may not be corrected through posture alone. Early diagnosis, careful monitoring, and targeted interventions are critical for preventing severe deformity, reducing pain, and preserving function. Understanding these underlying causes allows healthcare providers to tailor treatment to the individual's condition, age, and overall health.

Age And Lifestyle Influences On Kyphosis

Kyphosis is not solely the result of congenital or structural abnormalities. Both age and lifestyle factors play a critical role in the development, progression, and severity of spinal curvature. Understanding these influences can help individuals take proactive steps to maintain spinal health and prevent excessive curvature.

1. Age-Related Changes: As we age, natural changes in bone density, disc integrity, and muscle strength can contribute to kyphotic curvature. Key age-related factors include:

a. Osteoporosis:

- Reduced bone density weakens vertebrae, making them susceptible to compression fractures.
- Vertebral collapse increases thoracic curvature, often resulting in "dowager's hump" in older adults.

b. Degenerative Disc Disease:

- Intervertebral discs lose water content and flexibility with age.
- Loss of disc height alters spinal alignment and increases the risk of kyphotic curvature.

c. Muscle Weakness:

- Age-related decline in muscle mass (sarcopenia) weakens postural support in the back and core.
- Weak muscles fail to counteract gravitational forces, allowing the thoracic spine to round.

2. Lifestyle Factors: Daily habits and lifestyle choices can significantly influence spinal curvature over time. Common lifestyle-related contributors to kyphosis include:

a. Poor Posture:

- Slouching, forward head posture, and rounded shoulders increase thoracic curvature.
- Long-term poor posture, especially in adolescence or early adulthood, can become habitual and exacerbate kyphosis.

b. Sedentary Behavior:

- Extended sitting during work, study, or screen time weakens back muscles and promotes rounding of the upper back.
- Limited physical activity reduces flexibility and spinal stability.

c. Improper Lifting or Carrying Habits:

- Carrying heavy loads, particularly asymmetrically, strains the thoracic spine.
- Repeated poor lifting mechanics can reinforce curvature over time.

d. Lack of Exercise:

- Inadequate physical activity prevents strengthening of postural muscles.
- Stretching and mobility exercises are essential for counteracting age- and lifestyle-related changes.

3. Preventive and Corrective Measures: While age-related changes are inevitable, lifestyle adjustments can slow the progression of kyphosis and maintain spinal health:

- **Strength training** for back extensors, core muscles, and postural support.
- **Flexibility exercises** to stretch chest, shoulder, and spinal muscles.
- **Ergonomic adjustments** for workstations, seating, and daily routines.
- **Posture awareness** and periodic posture checks throughout the day.

- **Weight management and bone health strategies**, including adequate calcium and vitamin D intake.

Age and lifestyle factors interact to influence spinal curvature over time. Aging naturally weakens bones, discs, and muscles, making the spine more susceptible to kyphotic changes. Simultaneously, poor posture, sedentary habits, and lack of exercise can accelerate curvature and associated complications. By understanding these influences, individuals can adopt proactive measures — including exercise, posture correction, and ergonomic adjustments — to support spinal health, reduce progression, and improve quality of life.

CHAPTER THREE: DIAGNOSIS AND PROFESSIONAL GUIDANCE

Medical Assessment Of Kyphosis

Accurate assessment is crucial for diagnosing kyphosis, determining its type and severity, and guiding effective treatment. Medical evaluation combines **clinical examination, imaging studies, and functional assessments** to provide a comprehensive understanding of the spinal curvature.

1. Patient History: A thorough history provides essential context for understanding the origin and progression of kyphosis. Healthcare providers typically evaluate:

- **Age of onset:** Helps differentiate postural, Scheuermann's, congenital, or age-related kyphosis.
- **Progression:** Gradual versus rapid worsening may indicate underlying pathology.
- **Symptoms:** Pain, stiffness, fatigue, or neurological signs (numbness, tingling, weakness).
- **Lifestyle factors:** Posture habits, physical activity levels, and occupational demands.
- **Medical history:** Osteoporosis, trauma, spinal surgery, or systemic conditions affecting bones or muscles.

2. Physical Examination: Clinical evaluation focuses on posture, spinal flexibility, and muscular support. Key components include:

a. Visual Inspection:

- Observe the spine from the side to assess the thoracic curvature.
- Look for rounding of the upper back, forward head posture, or uneven shoulders/hips.

b. Palpation:

- Examine vertebrae and surrounding muscles for tenderness, tightness, or deformities.
- Identify areas of muscular imbalance or weakness contributing to postural kyphosis.

c. Flexibility and Range of Motion Tests:

- Determine whether the curvature is **flexible** (postural) or **rigid** (structural).
- Assess spinal mobility in forward bending, backward extension, and lateral flexion.

3. Imaging Studies: Imaging provides precise measurements of curvature and reveals structural abnormalities:

a. X-Rays:

- Standard method for measuring kyphotic angle using the **Cobb method**.
- Helps determine severity, vertebral shape, and alignment.

b. MRI (Magnetic Resonance Imaging):

- Evaluates soft tissues, intervertebral discs, spinal cord, and nerves.
- Used when neurological symptoms are present or structural abnormalities are suspected.

c. CT (Computed Tomography) Scan:

- Offers detailed visualization of bone structures.
- Useful in complex or congenital cases.

4. **Functional Assessments**: Medical assessment may also include evaluating the impact of kyphosis on function:

- **Gait and balance:** Severe curvature may alter walking mechanics.
- **Breathing tests:** Advanced thoracic kyphosis can limit lung expansion.
- **Muscle strength and endurance:** Weakness in postural muscles can indicate the need for targeted exercise interventions.

5. Classifying Severity: Kyphosis severity is commonly classified based on the **Cobb angle** measured on X-rays:

- **Mild:** 50°–60°
- **Moderate:** 60°–75°
- **Severe:** Greater than 75°

Severity classification guides treatment decisions, ranging from postural correction and exercise for mild cases to bracing or surgical intervention for severe structural kyphosis.

6. Early Detection Importance: Medical assessment is not only for diagnosing existing kyphosis but also for **early identification of progression**. Routine evaluations, especially during adolescence or in adults with osteoporosis, allow timely interventions to prevent worsening curvature, reduce pain, and preserve mobility.

The medical assessment of kyphosis involves a combination of **history-taking, physical examination, imaging studies, and functional evaluation**. By accurately identifying the type, severity, and underlying causes of kyphosis, healthcare providers can develop personalized treatment plans, optimize posture, and maintain spinal health over time.

Working With Healthcare Professionals

Managing kyphosis effectively often requires a **team-based approach** involving multiple healthcare professionals. Understanding each professional's role can help individuals receive the most appropriate care, ensure proper monitoring, and achieve the best outcomes.

1. Primary Care Physician (PCP): Your primary care physician is usually the first point of contact. They can:

- Evaluate initial concerns about posture, back pain, or spinal changes.
- Conduct basic physical examinations.
- Order initial imaging tests, such as X-rays.
- Refer patients to specialists for further evaluation or treatment.

2. Orthopedic Spine Specialist: Orthopedic surgeons who specialize in the spine are crucial for diagnosing and treating **structural kyphosis**. Their responsibilities include:

- Assessing severity and progression of the curvature.
- Determining whether surgical or non-surgical interventions are appropriate.
- Providing guidance on bracing, exercise programs, and rehabilitation.

3. Physical Therapist: Physical therapists play a central role in **postural correction and strengthening programs**. They can:

- Design personalized exercise regimens targeting the back, core, and chest muscles.
- Teach proper posture techniques for daily activities.
- Recommend stretches to improve spinal flexibility and reduce discomfort.
- Monitor progress and adjust programs as the patient's condition changes.

4. Occupational Therapist: Occupational therapists help patients adapt daily activities to **protect spinal health and maintain independence**. They may:

- Assess home, school, or workplace ergonomics.
- Recommend modifications to furniture, seating, or computer setup.
- Train patients in safe body mechanics for lifting, bending, or carrying objects.

5. Chiropractors (When Appropriate): Some individuals choose chiropractic care as part of their kyphosis management. Chiropractors may:

- Perform spinal mobilizations or adjustments to improve posture and alignment.
- Offer exercises and ergonomic advice to support spinal health. *Note:* Chiropractic care should be coordinated with medical professionals, particularly in cases of structural or severe kyphosis, osteoporosis, or spinal fractures.

6. Nutritionists or Dietitians: Bone and muscle health play a significant role in preventing kyphosis progression. Nutrition professionals can:

- Recommend diets rich in calcium, vitamin D, and protein to support bone strength.
- Advise on supplements when dietary intake is insufficient.
- Help maintain healthy weight to reduce stress on the spine.

7. Pain Management Specialists: In cases where kyphosis causes chronic discomfort, pain management specialists may:

- Prescribe medications for temporary relief.
- Offer minimally invasive procedures for pain control.
- Collaborate with therapists and physicians to develop a comprehensive pain management plan.

8. Collaborative Approach: Successful kyphosis management often depends on **coordinated care**. Key principles include:

- Regular communication among healthcare providers.

- Monitoring spinal curvature and functional changes over time.

- Adjusting treatment plans as the patient grows, ages, or experiences changes in health.

- Empowering patients with knowledge and exercises to maintain spinal health at home.

Working with healthcare professionals ensures that kyphosis is managed safely and effectively. From primary care physicians and orthopedic specialists to physical therapists, nutritionists, and pain management experts, a collaborative approach provides the best chance for maintaining posture, reducing discomfort, and preventing progression. Patients who actively participate in their care and communicate openly with their healthcare team achieve the most positive outcomes.

CHAPTER FOUR: CORRECTING POSTURE AND STRENGTHENING YOUR SPINE

Working With Healthcare Professionals

Managing kyphosis effectively often requires a **team-based approach** involving multiple healthcare professionals. Understanding each professional's role can help individuals receive the most appropriate care, ensure proper monitoring, and achieve the best outcomes.

1. Primary Care Physician (PCP): Your primary care physician is usually the first point of contact. They can:

- Evaluate initial concerns about posture, back pain, or spinal changes.
- Conduct basic physical examinations.
- Order initial imaging tests, such as X-rays.
- Refer patients to specialists for further evaluation or treatment.

2. Orthopedic Spine Specialist: Orthopedic surgeons who specialize in the spine are crucial for diagnosing and treating **structural kyphosis**. Their responsibilities include:

- Assessing severity and progression of the curvature.

- Determining whether surgical or non-surgical interventions are appropriate.
- Providing guidance on bracing, exercise programs, and rehabilitation.

3. Physical Therapist: Physical therapists play a central role in **postural correction and strengthening programs**. They can:

- Design personalized exercise regimens targeting the back, core, and chest muscles.
- Teach proper posture techniques for daily activities.
- Recommend stretches to improve spinal flexibility and reduce discomfort.
- Monitor progress and adjust programs as the patient's condition changes.

4. Occupational Therapist: Occupational therapists help patients adapt daily activities to **protect spinal health and maintain independence**. They may:

- Assess home, school, or workplace ergonomics.
- Recommend modifications to furniture, seating, or computer setup.
- Train patients in safe body mechanics for lifting, bending, or carrying objects.

5. Chiropractors (When Appropriate): Some individuals choose chiropractic care as part of their kyphosis management. Chiropractors may:

- Perform spinal mobilizations or adjustments to improve posture and alignment.
- Offer exercises and ergonomic advice to support spinal health. *Note:* Chiropractic care should be coordinated with medical professionals, particularly in cases of structural or severe kyphosis, osteoporosis, or spinal fractures.

6. Nutritionists or Dietitians: Bone and muscle health play a significant role in preventing kyphosis progression. Nutrition professionals can:

- Recommend diets rich in calcium, vitamin D, and protein to support bone strength.
- Advise on supplements when dietary intake is insufficient.
- Help maintain healthy weight to reduce stress on the spine.

7. Pain Management Specialists: In cases where kyphosis causes chronic discomfort, pain management specialists may:

- Prescribe medications for temporary relief.
- Offer minimally invasive procedures for pain control.

- Collaborate with therapists and physicians to develop a comprehensive pain management plan.

8. Collaborative Approach: Successful kyphosis management often depends on **coordinated care**. Key principles include:

- Regular communication among healthcare providers.
- Monitoring spinal curvature and functional changes over time.
- Adjusting treatment plans as the patient grows, ages, or experiences changes in health.
- Empowering patients with knowledge and exercises to maintain spinal health at home.

Working with healthcare professionals ensures that kyphosis is managed safely and effectively. From primary care physicians and orthopedic specialists to physical therapists, nutritionists, and pain management experts, a collaborative approach provides the best chance for maintaining posture, reducing discomfort, and preventing progression. Patients who actively participate in their care and communicate openly with their healthcare team achieve the most positive outcomes.

The Principles Of Postural Correction

Postural correction is a cornerstone in managing kyphosis, particularly for postural and mild structural forms. By improving alignment, strengthening supportive muscles, and maintaining spinal flexibility, individuals can reduce curvature progression, alleviate discomfort, and enhance overall function. The following principles provide a framework for effective postural correction.

1. Awareness of Posture: The first step in postural correction is **developing awareness** of how the spine is positioned throughout daily activities. Key practices include:

- Observing the alignment of the head, shoulders, and upper back in mirrors or photos.
- Noticing habitual slouching or forward head posture.
- Performing periodic "posture checks" during sitting, standing, or walking.
- Awareness allows individuals to consciously adjust posture and prevent the reinforcement of poor habits.

2. Strengthening Postural Muscles: Postural muscles are responsible for supporting the spine and maintaining proper curvature. Key areas to strengthen include:

- **Back extensors (erector spinae, multifidus):** Support thoracic and lumbar curves.

- **Core muscles (abdominals, obliques, transverse abdominis):** Stabilize the spine and pelvis.

- **Shoulder retractors (rhomboids, middle trapezius):** Counteract forward rounding of the shoulders.

Regular strength training helps counteract gravitational forces and reduces the tendency for the upper back to round.

3. Stretching Tight Muscles: Muscles that become shortened or tight contribute to forward rounding of the spine. Key stretches include:

- **Chest muscles (pectoralis major and minor):** Stretching these muscles opens the shoulders and chest.

- **Anterior shoulder and neck muscles:** Relieve tension from forward head posture.

- **Hip flexors:** Tight hips can indirectly affect spinal alignment.

Flexibility training complements strengthening exercises, allowing the spine to return to a neutral position more easily.

4. Maintaining Spinal Neutrality: Proper postural alignment involves maintaining the spine in a **neutral position**, preserving its natural curves:

- **Cervical lordosis:** Slight inward curve of the neck.

- **Thoracic kyphosis:** Gentle outward curve of the upper back.

- **Lumbar lordosis:** Mild inward curve of the lower back.

Neutral spine alignment reduces stress on vertebrae, discs, and ligaments while enhancing overall balance and movement efficiency.

5. Ergonomic and Environmental Adjustments: Postural correction is not limited to exercises. Daily environment and habits play a major role:

- Adjust chairs, desks, and screens to maintain upright posture.

- Use supportive seating and cushions to encourage spinal neutrality.

- Take regular breaks from sitting to stand, stretch, and move.

- Ensure proper lifting techniques and backpack weight distribution.

6. Consistency and Habit Formation: Effective postural correction requires consistent practice. Small, repeated adjustments over time can reshape habits and strengthen postural support. Strategies include:

- Setting reminders for posture checks.

- Integrating exercises into daily routines.

- Gradually increasing the difficulty and duration of strengthening and stretching programs.

7. Professional Guidance: While basic postural principles can be practiced independently, working with healthcare professionals enhances effectiveness:

- **Physical therapists** can design personalized exercise programs.
- **Occupational therapists** can optimize ergonomics at work or home.
- **Orthopedic specialists** can monitor structural kyphosis and provide corrective interventions if needed.

Postural correction is grounded in **awareness, muscle strengthening, stretching, spinal neutrality, ergonomic support, consistency, and professional guidance**. By applying these principles daily, individuals can improve alignment, reduce discomfort, prevent progression of kyphosis, and support long-term spinal health.

Stretching And Flexibility Exercises For Kyphosis

Stretching and flexibility exercises are essential components of kyphosis management. They help **lengthen tight muscles, improve spinal mobility, and counteract the forward rounding of the thoracic spine**. When combined with strengthening exercises and postural awareness, stretching contributes significantly to better posture and spinal health.

1. Chest (Pectoral) Stretch: Tight chest muscles pull the shoulders forward, increasing thoracic curvature. Stretching these muscles helps open the chest and align the shoulders.

Technique:

- Stand in a doorway or near a wall.
- Place your forearms on each side of the doorway at shoulder height.
- Step one foot forward and gently lean your chest through the doorway.
- Hold for **20–30 seconds**, repeat **2–3 times**.

2. Thoracic Extension Stretch: This exercise improves mobility in the upper back and counteracts rounding.

Technique:

- Sit or stand with your back straight.
- Interlace your fingers behind your head.
- Slowly lean back, extending the thoracic spine over a foam roller or rolled-up towel placed horizontally behind your upper back.
- Hold for **15–20 seconds**, repeat **2–3 times**.

3. Cat-Cow Stretch: The cat-cow sequence increases flexibility in the entire spine and relieves stiffness.

Technique:

Begin on hands and knees in a tabletop position.

- **Cat:** Round your back, tucking the chin toward your chest and drawing the belly in.
- **Cow:** Arch your back, lifting the head and tailbone toward the ceiling.
- Repeat **10–12 cycles**, moving slowly and with control.

4. Upper Back (Rhomboid) Stretch: Tight muscles between the shoulder blades can restrict mobility. Stretching them promotes thoracic extension and better posture.

Technique:

- Extend your arms in front of you, clasping your hands together.
- Push your hands forward while rounding the upper back slightly.
- Feel the stretch between your shoulder blades.
- Hold for **20–30 seconds**, repeat **2–3 times**.

5. Latissimus Dorsi Stretch: The lats connect the upper back to the lower spine; stretching them helps relieve tension and improve upper-body posture.

Technique:

- Kneel or stand and reach both arms overhead.
- Lean gently to one side, keeping arms straight.
- Hold for **20–30 seconds**, then switch sides.
- Repeat **2–3 times** per side.

6. Hip Flexor Stretch: Tight hip flexors can tilt the pelvis forward, indirectly affecting thoracic posture.

Technique:

- Step one foot forward into a lunge position.
- Keep the back leg straight and pelvis tucked slightly under.
- Push hips gently forward while keeping the upper body tall.
- Hold for **20–30 seconds**, repeat **2–3 times** per side.

7. Neck and Shoulder Stretch: Forward head posture often accompanies kyphosis. Stretching the neck and shoulders helps reduce tension.

Technique:

- Sit or stand upright.
- Tilt your head to one side, bringing the ear toward the shoulder.
- Use the hand on the same side to gently deepen the stretch.
- Hold for **15–20 seconds**, repeat **2–3 times** per side.

Tips for Effective Stretching

- Stretch **daily** for best results.

- Hold each stretch without bouncing; maintain steady breathing.

- Focus on feeling a gentle pull, not pain.

- Combine stretching with strengthening exercises for balanced postural correction.

- Use props such as foam rollers or resistance bands to enhance stretches when appropriate.

Stretching and flexibility exercises help **lengthen tight muscles, improve spinal mobility, and counteract kyphotic posture**. When practiced consistently and combined with strengthening and postural training, these exercises support spinal health, reduce discomfort, and improve overall posture.

Strengthening And Stabilization Exercises For Kyphosis

Strengthening and stabilization exercises are essential for correcting and preventing kyphosis. While stretching addresses tight muscles, **strengthening exercises target weak postural muscles**, helping maintain proper spinal alignment, improve posture, and reduce discomfort. Emphasis is placed on the **back, core, and shoulder muscles**, which provide structural support to the spine.

1. Wall Angels: Wall angels strengthen the upper back and shoulder muscles while promoting thoracic extension.

Technique:

- Stand with your back against a wall, feet slightly away, and lower back gently pressed to the wall.
- Place your arms against the wall in a "goalpost" position (elbows bent at 90°).
- Slowly slide your arms upward as if making a snow angel, then return to the starting position.
- Repeat **10–15 times**, 2–3 sets.

2. Prone Back Extensions: This exercise targets the **erector spinae and mid-back muscles**, strengthening spinal extensors.

Technique:

- Lie face down on a mat with arms at your sides or behind your head.
- Gently lift your chest and upper torso off the floor without straining your neck.
- Hold for **3–5 seconds**, then lower slowly.

- Repeat **10–12 times**, 2–3 sets.

3. Rows (Resistance Band or Dumbbell): Rows strengthen the **rhomboids and middle trapezius**, helping retract the shoulders and reduce rounding.

Technique:

- Hold a resistance band or dumbbells with arms extended in front.
- Pull the band or weights toward your chest, squeezing shoulder blades together.
- Slowly return to the starting position.
- Repeat **12–15 times**, 2–3 sets.

4. Plank Variations: Planks stabilize the **core muscles**, including abdominals and spinal stabilizers, supporting proper posture.

Technique:

- Start in a forearm plank position, elbows under shoulders, body in a straight line.
- Engage your core and hold for **20–60 seconds**.
- Gradually increase duration as strength improves.
- Variations include side planks and planks with leg lifts for additional challenge.

5. Bird-Dog Exercise: The bird-dog strengthens the **lower back, glutes, and core**, promoting spinal stability.

Technique:

- Begin on hands and knees, elbows under shoulders, knees under hips.
- Extend your right arm forward and left leg backward simultaneously, keeping your spine neutral.
- Hold for **3–5 seconds**, then return to start.
- Repeat with opposite arm and leg.
- Perform **10–12 repetitions per side**, 2–3 sets.

6. Shoulder Blade Squeeze: This simple exercise improves **postural endurance** by activating muscles that retract and stabilize the shoulders.

Technique:

- Sit or stand upright with arms at your sides.
- Squeeze shoulder blades together and hold for **5–10 seconds**.
- Release slowly.
- Repeat **10–15 times**, 2–3 sets.

7. Dead Bug Exercise: Dead bugs strengthen the **deep core muscles**, which support spinal alignment and posture.

Technique:

- Lie on your back with arms extended toward the ceiling and knees bent at 90°.
- Slowly lower your right arm and left leg toward the floor while keeping your lower back pressed to the mat.
- Return to start and switch sides.
- Repeat **10–12 times per side**, 2–3 sets.

Tips for Effective Strengthening:

- Perform exercises **3–4 times per week** for optimal results.
- Focus on **controlled movements** and proper form to prevent strain.
- Combine strengthening with **stretching and postural training** for balanced improvement.
- Progress gradually, increasing resistance or repetitions as strength improves.
- Seek professional guidance if you have **structural kyphosis or pain**.

Strengthening and stabilization exercises target weak postural muscles, support the spine, and counteract kyphotic curvature. When performed consistently and paired with flexibility and postural awareness, these exercises can **improve posture, reduce discomfort, and prevent progression of kyphosis**, promoting long-term spinal health.

Balance And Movement Training For Kyphosis

Balance and movement training are critical components in managing kyphosis. Proper spinal alignment depends not only on muscle strength and flexibility but also on **coordination, balance, and body awareness**. Training these skills helps prevent falls, improve posture, and enhance functional mobility, particularly in older adults or individuals with advanced curvature.

1. Importance of Balance Training: Kyphosis alters the body's center of gravity, often causing a forward lean. This can lead to:

- Increased risk of falls and injuries
- Fatigue and instability during standing or walking
- Compensatory movement patterns that worsen curvature
- Balance training strengthens **stabilizing muscles**, improves proprioception (awareness of body position), and enhances overall stability.

2. Core Stabilization for Balance: A strong core provides a stable foundation for spinal alignment and movement.

Exercises include:

a. Standing Marches:

- Stand upright with feet hip-width apart.
- Lift one knee toward the chest while keeping your torso tall.
- Alternate legs slowly, maintaining balance.
- Perform **10–15 repetitions per side**, 2–3 sets.

b. Single-Leg Stands:

- Stand near a wall or chair for support if needed.
- Lift one foot off the ground and balance on the other leg.
- Hold for **15–30 seconds**, then switch sides.
- Repeat **2–3 times per leg**.

3. **Dynamic Movement and Coordination**: Dynamic exercises improve **functional mobility** and reinforce proper posture during daily activities:

a. Heel-to-Toe Walk:

- Walk in a straight line, placing the heel of one foot directly in front of the toes of the other foot.
- Keep the torso upright and shoulders relaxed.
- Perform for **10–20 steps**, repeat 2–3 times.

b. Arm and Leg Coordination

- Stand tall with feet hip-width apart.
- Extend opposite arm and leg forward and backward, maintaining spinal neutrality.
- Return to start and switch sides.
- Repeat **10–12 times per side**, 2–3 sets.

4. **Functional Movement Integration**: Incorporating balance and movement into daily activities enhances spinal stability:

- Use **stairs** to practice controlled, upright movement.
- Carry objects with proper posture to reinforce spinal alignment.
- Practice **reaching and bending** with the core engaged, avoiding slouching or rounding the back.

5. **Mind-Body Techniques**: Activities that combine movement, balance, and body awareness can improve posture and reduce kyphosis-related discomfort:

- **Yoga:** Focus on spinal extension, balance poses, and deep breathing.
- **Tai Chi:** Enhances coordination, stability, and controlled movement.
- **Pilates:** Strengthens the core and improves postural control through precise movements.

6. Tips for Safe and Effective Balance Training

- Start with **assisted or supported exercises** if you are unstable.

- Progress gradually to more challenging positions or dynamic movements.

- Perform exercises **3–4 times per week** for consistent improvement.

- Combine balance training with **strengthening, stretching, and postural correction** for optimal results.

- Consult a healthcare professional if you have **structural kyphosis, osteoporosis, or a history of falls**.

Balance and movement training strengthen stabilizing muscles, enhance body awareness, and improve coordination. By integrating these exercises into a comprehensive kyphosis management plan, individuals can **maintain spinal alignment, prevent falls, and support functional mobility**, contributing to long-term spinal health and improved quality of life.

CHAPTER FIVE: LIFESTYLE INTEGRATION FOR PERMANENT IMPROVEMENT

Ergonomics And Workstation Setup

Proper ergonomics are essential for preventing and managing kyphosis, especially in today's world of prolonged sitting, computer use, and screen time.

A well-designed workstation supports spinal alignment, reduces muscle strain, and encourages healthy posture throughout the day.

1. Chair Selection and Positioning: A supportive chair is the foundation of good workstation ergonomics:

- **Seat height:** Adjust so feet are flat on the floor and knees are at a 90° angle.
- **Lumbar support:** Use built-in or external lumbar support to maintain the natural curve of the lower back.
- **Seat depth:** Ensure there is 2–3 inches of space between the back of the knees and the seat edge.
- **Armrests:** Adjust to allow relaxed shoulders and elbows close to the body at a 90° angle.

2. Desk Height and Layout: Desk positioning influences spinal posture and comfort:

- **Height:** Place the desk so elbows remain at approximately 90° while typing.
- **Surface organization:** Keep frequently used items within easy reach to avoid leaning forward.

Monitor placement:

- Top of the screen should be at or slightly below eye level.
- Maintain a distance of 20–30 inches (50–75 cm) from the eyes.
- Center the monitor directly in front to avoid twisting the neck.

3. Keyboard and Mouse Positioning: Proper placement reduces forward rounding and shoulder strain:

- Keep the keyboard and mouse close enough to avoid reaching.
- Maintain wrists in a neutral position, avoiding excessive flexion or extension.
- Consider ergonomic keyboards or mouse designs to reduce strain.

4. Foot Support:

- Use a footrest if feet do not comfortably reach the floor.
- Keep weight evenly distributed on both feet while seated.

5. Movement and Breaks: Even with optimal workstation setup, prolonged sitting can exacerbate kyphosis:

- Stand up and move every 30–45 minutes.
- Perform **short stretches** for the chest, back, and shoulders during breaks.
- Incorporate **micro-movements** such as shoulder rolls or spinal extensions to counteract rounding.

6. Ergonomic Accessories: Additional tools can enhance spinal alignment and comfort:

- **Lumbar cushions** or rolled towels for lower back support.
- **Adjustable monitor stands** to achieve eye-level positioning.
- **Sit-stand desks** for alternating between sitting and standing.
- **Anti-fatigue mats** for standing positions to reduce strain on legs and lower back.

7. Home and Remote Work Considerations:

- Ensure laptops, tablets, and other devices are positioned to minimize forward head posture.
- Avoid working from couches or beds for extended periods.
- Set up dedicated workstations even in small spaces to support proper posture consistently.

Ergonomics and workstation setup play a vital role in **preventing postural kyphosis and minimizing discomfort**. By choosing supportive chairs, arranging desks and monitors correctly, maintaining proper keyboard and mouse positioning, and incorporating regular movement, individuals can reduce spinal strain, maintain alignment, and support long-term spinal health.

Daily Habits That Improve Posture

Maintaining good posture throughout the day is essential for preventing the progression of kyphosis and reducing discomfort. Small, consistent habits can make a significant difference in spinal health, complementing exercises, stretching, and ergonomic adjustments.

1. Mindful Sitting:

- Keep your **back straight** and shoulders relaxed while sitting.
- Keep **feet flat** on the floor and knees at a 90° angle.
- Use **lumbar support** to maintain the natural curve of the lower back.
- Avoid crossing legs for long periods, which can create pelvic imbalance.

2. Proper Standing Posture:

- Stand tall with **weight evenly distributed** on both feet.
- Keep **shoulders relaxed** and aligned with the hips.
- Engage **core muscles** gently to support the spine.
- Avoid locking knees or slouching while standing for extended periods.

3. Walking and Movement Awareness

- Walk with your **head up**, looking forward rather than downward.
- Keep **shoulders back** and spine elongated.
- Swing arms naturally to support balance and posture.
- Incorporate walking breaks throughout sedentary periods.

4. Lifting and Carrying Safely:

- Bend at the **knees and hips**, not the waist, when lifting objects.
- Keep objects **close to the body** to reduce spinal stress.
- Avoid twisting while lifting; pivot with your feet instead.
- For backpacks, distribute weight evenly on both shoulders and avoid overloading.

5. Sleeping Habits:

- Use a **supportive mattress** that maintains spinal alignment.
- Choose pillows that support the **neck without overextending** it.

- Sleeping on your back with a small pillow under the knees or on your side with a pillow between the knees can promote spinal neutrality.

- Avoid stomach sleeping, which can increase thoracic rounding.

6. Regular Micro-Breaks:

- Take short breaks every **30–60 minutes** to stand, stretch, or move.

- Perform simple stretches for the **chest, shoulders, and upper back** during breaks.

- Use these breaks as reminders to **check and correct posture**.

7. Strengthening Everyday Movements:

- Integrate **postural exercises into daily routines**, such as shoulder blade squeezes while waiting in line.

- Engage core muscles when bending, lifting, or reaching.

- Practice **spinal elongation** exercises during routine activities like brushing teeth or cooking.

8. Technology Use:

- Position **screens at eye level** to avoid forward head posture.

- Hold smartphones and tablets at **eye height**, not on the lap.

- Limit prolonged device use and incorporate breaks to stretch and reset posture.

9. Awareness and Habit Formation:

- Regularly **check posture in mirrors** or use posture reminders on your phone.

- Reinforce positive posture with cues like "shoulders back and down" or "spine tall."

- Over time, these micro-adjustments become natural, reducing the likelihood of kyphosis progression.

Daily habits—ranging from mindful sitting and standing to safe lifting, proper sleep, and regular movement—are vital for **supporting spinal alignment and improving posture**. When practiced consistently, these habits complement exercises, stretching, and ergonomic strategies, helping to **prevent progression of kyphosis, reduce pain, and enhance overall spinal health**.

Nutrition For Spinal Health

Proper nutrition plays a critical role in maintaining strong bones, supporting muscle function, and preventing conditions that can exacerbate kyphosis. A diet that provides essential vitamins, minerals, and macronutrients helps preserve spinal integrity and overall musculoskeletal health.

1. Calcium: Building Strong Bones: Calcium is vital for bone density and strength, helping prevent vertebral compression fractures that can worsen kyphosis.

Sources:

- Dairy products: milk, yogurt, cheese
- Leafy greens: kale, bok choy, spinach
- Fortified foods: plant-based milk, cereals
- Fish with soft bones: sardines, salmon

Tip: Pair calcium with **vitamin D** to enhance absorption.

2. Vitamin D: Supporting Calcium Absorption: Vitamin D is essential for calcium absorption and bone mineralization. Low levels can increase fracture risk.

Sources:

- Sunlight exposure (10–20 minutes daily)
- Fatty fish: salmon, mackerel, tuna
- Egg yolks
- Fortified foods: milk, orange juice, cereals

3. Protein: Supporting Muscles and Connective Tissue: Adequate protein intake strengthens **postural muscles and connective tissues** that support the spine.

Sources:

- Lean meats: chicken, turkey, beef
- Fish and seafood
- Eggs
- Legumes: beans, lentils, chickpeas
- Nuts and seeds

Tip: Spread protein intake throughout the day for optimal muscle repair and growth.

4. Magnesium and Potassium: Bone and Muscle Health: Magnesium and potassium contribute to **bone density, nerve function, and muscle contraction**, helping maintain spinal stability.

Sources of Magnesium:

- Nuts and seeds: almonds, pumpkin seeds
- Whole grains: brown rice, oats, quinoa
- Leafy greens: spinach, Swiss chard

Sources of Potassium:

- Bananas, oranges, and avocados
- Sweet potatoes and potatoes
- Beans and lentils

5. Omega-3 Fatty Acids: Reducing Inflammation: Omega-3 fatty acids support joint health and may reduce inflammation associated with spinal discomfort.

Sources:

- Fatty fish: salmon, mackerel, sardines
- Flaxseeds and chia seeds
- Walnuts

6. Antioxidants and Vitamins C & K: Antioxidants and vitamins like C and K promote **collagen formation** and bone strength:

- **Vitamin C:** citrus fruits, berries, bell peppers, broccoli
- **Vitamin K:** kale, spinach, Brussels sprouts

Collagen is a key component of spinal discs, ligaments, and connective tissue, helping maintain flexibility and integrity.

7. Hydration: Adequate water intake supports **intervertebral disc health** and overall muscle function:

- Aim for at least **6–8 cups of water daily**, adjusting for activity level and climate.
- Hydrated discs maintain flexibility and reduce risk of degeneration.

8. Limiting Harmful Substances:

- **Excess sugar and processed foods** may increase inflammation and reduce nutrient density.
- **Excess caffeine and alcohol** can reduce calcium absorption, weakening bones.
- **Smoking** impairs bone health and tissue repair, increasing the risk of kyphotic progression.

9. Practical Tips for Spinal Nutrition:

- Include **bone-supporting nutrients** in every meal.
- Consider **fortified foods or supplements** if dietary intake is insufficient, after consulting a healthcare professional.
- Pair nutrient-rich foods with **regular exercise** to maximize musculoskeletal health.

Nutrition is a foundational aspect of spinal health, supporting **bone density, muscle strength, and connective tissue integrity**. A diet rich in calcium, vitamin D, protein, magnesium, potassium, and omega-3 fatty acids, combined with proper hydration and avoidance of harmful substances, can **help prevent kyphosis progression, reduce discomfort, and maintain spinal function throughout life**.

Tracking Your Progress

Monitoring your posture and spinal health over time is essential for managing kyphosis effectively. Tracking progress allows you to **measure improvements, identify areas that need more attention, and stay motivated**. Both subjective observations and objective measurements play a role in assessing your posture, strength, flexibility, and overall spinal well-being.

1. Posture Self-Assessment: Regularly observing your posture helps identify changes in curvature and alignment:

- **Mirror checks:** Stand sideways in front of a full-length mirror and observe your head, shoulders, and upper back alignment.
- **Photo documentation:** Take photos from multiple angles weekly or monthly to visually track changes.
- **Posture journals:** Note daily habits, exercises completed, and any pain or stiffness experienced.

2. Measuring Spinal Curvature: For a more objective assessment:

- **Cobb angle measurement:** Performed by a healthcare professional via X-rays for precise spinal curvature tracking.
- **Inclinometer or smartphone apps:** Some tools allow rough estimates of thoracic curvature at home.

- **Tape measures or plumb lines:** Can be used to track changes in shoulder or upper back rounding over time.

3. **Strength and Flexibility Tracking**: Record improvements in muscular strength and flexibility to gauge functional progress:

- **Strength tests:** Track repetitions, resistance levels, or duration of exercises like planks, rows, or wall angels.
- **Flexibility tests:** Measure progress in stretches, such as chest opening, thoracic extension, or hamstring flexibility.
- **Balance tests:** Monitor stability through single-leg stands, heel-to-toe walking, or other balance exercises.

4. **Symptom Monitoring**: Pay attention to changes in physical sensations:

- **Pain levels:** Track frequency, intensity, and location of discomfort.
- **Fatigue or stiffness:** Note any improvements or worsening throughout the day.
- **Functionality:** Observe ease of movement, posture maintenance, and breathing capacity.

5. **Setting Realistic Goals**: Tracking allows you to establish **short-term and long-term goals**:

- **Short-term goals:** Completing exercises consistently, improving flexibility, or reducing pain during daily activities.
- **Long-term goals:** Achieving measurable improvements in spinal alignment, strength, and posture habits.

6. Using Technology: Technology can assist in tracking posture and progress:

- **Posture tracking apps:** Provide reminders, real-time posture feedback, and historical data.
- **Fitness trackers or smartwatches:** Monitor movement, activity levels, and exercise adherence.
- **Video analysis:** Record and analyze exercise form and posture correction techniques.

7. Professional Monitoring: Regular check-ins with healthcare professionals can provide:

- Accurate measurements of spinal curvature.
- Feedback on exercise technique and effectiveness.
- Adjustments to treatment plans based on progress.

8. Celebrating Milestones: Acknowledging small achievements helps maintain motivation:

- Improved posture during daily activities.

- Increased strength, flexibility, or balance.

- Reduction in pain or discomfort.

- Successful integration of ergonomic and lifestyle changes.

Tracking your progress in posture, spinal alignment, strength, flexibility, and overall well-being is essential for **managing kyphosis effectively**. By combining self-assessment, objective measurements, symptom monitoring, goal setting, and professional feedback, individuals can maintain motivation, adjust strategies as needed, and achieve long-term improvements in spinal health and posture.

CHAPTER SIX: SPECIAL SITUATIONS AND ADVANCED CONSIDERATIONS

Kyphosis In Children And Adolescents

Kyphosis can affect individuals of all ages, but its onset in **childhood and adolescence** requires special attention. During these formative years, the spine is still developing, and early detection, intervention, and monitoring can prevent progression and minimize long-term complications.

1. Common Types in Young Individuals: Several types of kyphosis are more prevalent in children and adolescents:

Postural Kyphosis:

- Most common in teenagers.
- Often linked to slouching or poor posture habits.
- Usually flexible and rarely causes pain.

Scheuermann's Kyphosis:

- A structural condition where vertebrae grow unevenly, creating a rigid curve.
- Typically appears during adolescence, especially in boys aged 12–16.
- Can cause mild back pain and noticeable spinal rounding.

Congenital Kyphosis:

- Present at birth due to vertebral malformations.
- Can progress rapidly if untreated, sometimes requiring early surgical intervention.

2. **Signs and Symptoms**: Parents, teachers, and healthcare providers should watch for:

- Rounded upper back or noticeable hump.
- Forward head posture or uneven shoulders.
- Fatigue or discomfort during prolonged sitting or physical activity.
- Limited spinal flexibility in structural cases.
- Early detection allows for interventions that can **correct or control curvature** before it worsens.

3. **Importance of Early Assessment**: Early evaluation by a pediatrician or orthopedic specialist is critical:

- Physical exams and posture observation help differentiate **flexible postural kyphosis** from **structural forms** like Scheuermann's.
- Imaging (X-rays) may be used to measure spinal curvature and monitor progression.

- Identifying rapid progression or severe curvature early can prevent future complications.

4. Treatment Approaches in Children and Adolescents: Treatment strategies depend on the type, severity, and age of the child:

Postural Kyphosis:

- Encouraged through postural education and exercises to strengthen the back and core muscles.
- Physical therapy can improve flexibility and postural awareness.

Scheuermann's Kyphosis:

- Mild cases may benefit from exercises and physical therapy.
- Moderate to severe curves may require **bracing** during growth periods to slow progression.
- Rarely, surgery is considered for severe, rigid curves.

Congenital Kyphosis:

- Often requires **early surgical intervention** due to risk of rapid progression.
- Regular monitoring and follow-up are essential.

5. Lifestyle and Supportive Strategies

- Encourage **regular physical activity** that strengthens back and core muscles.
- Promote **ergonomic seating** for schoolwork and study.
- Avoid prolonged slouching during screen time or reading.
- Educate children about **spinal health** and posture from an early age.

6. Monitoring and Follow-Up: Children and adolescents with kyphosis require ongoing monitoring:

- Regular clinical check-ups to assess growth and curvature changes.
- Imaging as recommended by healthcare professionals to track progression.
- Adjustment of exercises, braces, or other interventions based on growth and spinal development.

7. Psychological Considerations: Kyphosis in young individuals can affect **self-esteem and body image**, particularly during adolescence:

- Support from parents, teachers, and peers is important.
- Encourage participation in physical activities that promote confidence and strength.

- Counseling or support groups may be helpful for adolescents struggling with appearance or social concerns.

Kyphosis in children and adolescents requires **early recognition, careful monitoring, and tailored interventions**. By identifying postural versus structural types, applying appropriate exercises or bracing, and supporting spinal health through lifestyle habits, parents and healthcare providers can **help young individuals maintain proper posture, prevent progression, and promote both physical and emotional well-being**.

Kyphosis In Older Adults

Kyphosis is particularly common in older adults due to age-related changes in bone density, muscle strength, and spinal structure. Understanding its causes, consequences, and management strategies is essential to maintaining mobility, independence, and quality of life in later years.

1. Age-Related Causes: Several factors contribute to kyphosis in older adults:

- **Osteoporosis:** Weakens vertebrae, increasing the risk of compression fractures that worsen spinal curvature.

- **Degenerative Disc Disease:** Discs lose height and elasticity, leading to increased thoracic rounding.
- **Muscle Weakness:** Decline in back extensor and core muscle strength reduces postural support.
- **Postural Habits:** Long-term slouching or sedentary lifestyle can exacerbate curvature over time.

2. **Signs and Symptoms**: Kyphosis in older adults may present as:

- Noticeable forward rounding of the upper back ("dowager's hump").
- Loss of height over time.
- Back pain or stiffness.
- Reduced mobility and difficulty performing daily activities.
- Balance issues, increasing fall risk.

3. **Health Implications**: Severe kyphosis in older adults can affect:

- **Respiratory function:** Reduced lung capacity due to thoracic compression.
- **Digestive health:** Compression of abdominal organs may lead to discomfort or reduced appetite.
- **Balance and mobility:** Forward-leaning posture increases fall risk.

- **Quality of life:** Pain, reduced independence, and self-image concerns.

4. Assessment and Monitoring: Older adults should have regular assessments to monitor spinal health:

- Physical examination to assess curvature, flexibility, and balance.
- Imaging (X-rays, bone density scans) to evaluate vertebral integrity.
- Review of risk factors such as osteoporosis or prior fractures.

5. Non-Surgical Management: For most older adults, non-surgical approaches are first-line strategies:

Exercise and Strengthening:

- Focus on back extensors, core muscles, and postural muscles.
- Include balance and flexibility training to reduce fall risk.

Postural Awareness:

- Practice proper alignment during sitting, standing, and walking.
- Use supportive seating and pillows as needed.

Bracing (if indicated):

- Lightweight thoracic braces may provide temporary support and pain relief in some cases.

Nutrition:

- Adequate calcium, vitamin D, and protein intake to support bone and muscle health.

6. Surgical Considerations: Surgery may be considered in older adults with:

- Severe, progressive curvature causing pain or functional impairment.
- Spinal fractures that cannot be managed conservatively.
- Neurological symptoms resulting from spinal cord or nerve compression.
- Surgical planning in older adults must account for **bone quality, comorbidities, and overall health**.

7. Lifestyle and Daily Strategies:

- Encourage **regular physical activity**, tailored to ability and safety.
- Maintain **ergonomic seating** at home to support spinal alignment.
- Implement **fall prevention strategies**, including safe footwear, handrails, and adequate lighting.
- Practice **breathing exercises** to maximize lung capacity.

8. Psychological and Social Support: Kyphosis can affect self-esteem and independence:

- Encourage social engagement and activities that build confidence.
- Offer emotional support and counseling if needed.
- Educate family and caregivers on proper support techniques for daily activities.

Kyphosis in older adults is often a **multifactorial condition** influenced by osteoporosis, muscle weakness, and degenerative changes. Through **early assessment, exercise, postural correction, nutrition, and supportive strategies**, older adults can maintain mobility, reduce pain, prevent progression, and preserve independence and quality of life. In severe cases, surgical interventions may be appropriate, but conservative management remains the primary approach for most individuals.

Combining Medical And Natural Approaches For Kyphosis

Managing kyphosis effectively often requires a **multifaceted approach**, blending medical treatments with natural, lifestyle-based strategies. This combination addresses both the **structural aspects of the spine** and the **muscular, postural, and lifestyle factors** that influence curvature and spinal health.

1. Understanding the Complementary Roles

Medical Interventions:

- Focus on addressing structural causes, pain, or complications.
- Include medications for pain or osteoporosis, bracing, and surgical options when necessary.
- Provide precise diagnosis and monitoring through imaging and specialist evaluation.

Natural and Lifestyle Approaches:

- Target posture, muscle strength, flexibility, and overall wellness.
- Include exercises, stretching, ergonomic adjustments, nutrition, and mindfulness techniques.
- Help prevent further curvature progression and support daily function.

2. Integrating Exercise with Medical Guidance:

- **Physical therapy programs** can be tailored to both structural and postural kyphosis, complementing medical interventions.
- Core, back, and shoulder strengthening exercises improve stability, even for those using braces or recovering from surgery.

- Stretching routines reduce muscle tightness and improve spinal mobility, supporting medical treatment outcomes.

3. Bracing and Natural Support:

- Braces are often prescribed to slow progression, especially in adolescents or severe cases.
- Combining bracing with **postural exercises** enhances effectiveness:
- Muscles remain active while supported, preventing atrophy.
- Encourages proper alignment even when the brace is not worn.

4. Nutrition and Bone Health: Medical management of osteoporosis or bone density issues can include **medications such as bisphosphonates**, while natural approaches focus on:

Calcium and vitamin D intake:

- Adequate protein for muscle support
- Anti-inflammatory nutrients (omega-3 fatty acids, antioxidants)
- This combination strengthens bones and supports overall musculoskeletal health.

5. Pain Management:

- Medical options: medications, injections, or surgical interventions for severe cases.

- Natural strategies: gentle exercises, stretching, yoga, and mindfulness techniques can reduce pain and improve mobility without over-reliance on drugs.

6. Lifestyle and Ergonomics Integration:

- Medical advice often emphasizes avoiding certain activities or movements that exacerbate curvature.
- Natural approaches teach **safe movement patterns, ergonomic setups, and daily posture habits** to maintain spinal health.
- Combining both ensures **prevention of injury** and **enhancement of functional mobility**.

7. Mind-Body Practices: Techniques such as **yoga, Pilates, Tai Chi, and mindfulness exercises** can complement medical treatments by:

- Improving spinal flexibility
- Enhancing balance and coordination
- Reducing stress-related muscle tension

These practices support both physical recovery and mental well-being.

8. Monitoring and Adjustment: Combining approaches requires **ongoing assessment**:

- Track posture, strength, flexibility, and pain levels.

- Adjust exercises and interventions based on medical recommendations and personal progress.
- Regular check-ups with healthcare professionals ensure safe and effective integration.

A **holistic approach** to kyphosis management combines medical treatments with natural, lifestyle-based strategies. By integrating **physical therapy, bracing, nutrition, exercise, ergonomic practices, and mind-body techniques**, individuals can:

- Reduce pain and discomfort
- Improve posture and spinal stability
- Prevent progression of curvature
- Enhance overall quality of life

This integrated strategy addresses **both the structural and functional aspects of kyphosis**, providing the most effective long-term outcomes.

Frequently Asked Questions (Faqs) About Kyphosis And Spinal Health

1. **What is kyphosis?** Kyphosis is an excessive forward curvature of the thoracic (upper) spine, resulting in a rounded upper back. Mild kyphosis is often normal, but severe curvature can cause pain, reduced mobility, and postural issues.

2. How is normal spinal curvature different from kyphosis? Normal thoracic curvature ranges from **20° to 45°**. Kyphosis occurs when this curve exceeds normal limits, often over 50°, creating a visible hump and potential structural and functional problems.

3. What are the common types of kyphosis?

- **Postural Kyphosis:** Caused by poor posture; usually flexible and non-structural.
- **Scheuermann's Kyphosis:** Structural, seen in adolescents due to uneven vertebral growth.
- **Congenital Kyphosis:** Present at birth from vertebral malformations.
- **Osteoporotic Kyphosis:** Age-related, caused by vertebral fractures from weakened bones.

4. What causes kyphosis in children? Common causes include postural habits, Scheuermann's disease, or congenital vertebral anomalies. Rapid growth during adolescence can exacerbate structural curvature.

5. What causes kyphosis in older adults? Osteoporosis, degenerative disc disease, muscle weakness, and long-term postural habits contribute to kyphosis in older adults. Vertebral compression fractures are also a common factor.

6. Can kyphosis be prevented? Mild postural kyphosis can often be prevented by maintaining good posture, strengthening postural muscles, practicing spinal exercises, and following proper ergonomics from an early age.

7. What are the signs of kyphosis?

- Rounded upper back or hump
- Forward head posture
- Uneven shoulders or hips
- Back pain or stiffness
- Reduced flexibility and mobility

8. How is kyphosis diagnosed? Diagnosis includes physical examination, posture assessment, medical history, and imaging studies like X-rays to measure spinal curvature (Cobb angle).

9. Is kyphosis painful? Postural kyphosis is usually painless. Structural or severe kyphosis may cause chronic back pain, stiffness, fatigue, or nerve-related symptoms.

10. How does kyphosis affect daily life? Severe kyphosis can limit mobility, reduce endurance, affect balance, impair breathing, and impact self-esteem due to appearance concerns.

11. Can exercises correct kyphosis? Yes. Postural exercises, stretching, core and back strengthening, and balance training can **improve spinal alignment, reduce pain, and prevent progression**, particularly for postural and mild Scheuermann's kyphosis.

12. What types of exercises are recommended?

- Wall angels, chin tucks, cat-cow stretches
- Thoracic extensions and bird-dog exercises
- Core strengthening (planks, seated marches)
- Shoulder blade squeezes and resistance band rows
- Balance exercises (single-leg stands, heel-to-toe walking)

13. Can kyphosis be treated with physical therapy alone? Mild to moderate postural or Scheuermann's kyphosis often responds well to **physical therapy**. Severe structural kyphosis may require additional interventions like bracing or surgery.

14. When is surgery needed for kyphosis? Surgery is usually considered for:

- Severe curvature causing pain or functional impairment
- Progressive curves not responding to conservative therapy
- Neurological symptoms due to spinal cord compression
- Congenital kyphosis with rapid progression

15. How effective is bracing for kyphosis? Bracing is most effective for **adolescents with structural curves** and during periods of growth. It can slow progression and improve alignment when combined with exercises.

16. Can kyphosis worsen over time? Yes, untreated structural or severe postural kyphosis can progress, especially during periods of growth or with age-related bone loss and muscle weakening.

17. How does posture influence kyphosis? Slouching, forward head posture, and weak postural muscles can lead to postural kyphosis and exacerbate existing curvature. Proper posture is essential for prevention and management.

18. Can nutrition affect spinal health? Yes. Adequate intake of **calcium, vitamin D, protein, magnesium, and antioxidants** supports bone density, muscle strength, and connective tissue integrity, reducing the risk of kyphosis progression.

19. Are there lifestyle changes that help kyphosis?

- Maintain good posture at work, home, and during activities
- Use ergonomic furniture and devices
- Perform regular stretching, strengthening, and balance exercises
- Avoid prolonged slouching and sedentary behavior
- Engage in physical activity for bone and muscle health

20. Can kyphosis affect breathing? Severe thoracic curvature can compress the chest cavity, reducing lung capacity and making deep breathing more difficult. Exercises that **open the chest and strengthen back muscles** can improve respiratory function.

21. How can kyphosis impact balance and fall risk? Forward curvature shifts the center of gravity, reducing stability. Strengthening postural and core muscles, along with balance exercises, can reduce fall risk.

22. Is kyphosis hereditary? Scheuermann's disease and some congenital kyphosis forms may have a **genetic component**, but postural and osteoporotic kyphosis are influenced more by lifestyle and bone health.

23. How can I monitor kyphosis at home?

- Use mirrors or photos to track spinal alignment
- Keep a posture journal or log exercises and pain
- Use posture-tracking apps or simple plumb-line tests
- Regularly compare progress to baseline observations

24. Can kyphosis cause nerve issues? Severe structural curvature or vertebral fractures can compress spinal nerves, leading to **numbness, tingling, or weakness in the limbs**. Prompt medical evaluation is necessary.

25. Are there exercises that should be avoided?

- High-impact activities or heavy lifting without proper form may worsen curvature.
- Overextending the thoracic spine without guidance can increase risk of injury.
- Always consult a healthcare professional before starting new exercises if curvature is severe.

26. Can children with postural kyphosis fully recover? Yes. With **early intervention, exercise, and postural awareness**, children with postural kyphosis can often achieve normal spinal alignment and prevent progression.

27. How long does it take to see improvement? Mild postural improvements may appear in **4–6 weeks** with consistent exercises and daily posture habits. Structural improvement may take months, and some severe cases require ongoing management.

28. Can kyphosis be reversed?

- **Postural kyphosis:** Often reversible with proper exercise and habits.
- **Structural kyphosis (Scheuermann's or congenital):** Cannot always be fully reversed, but progression can be minimized, and posture can improve with therapy and bracing.

29. How does age affect kyphosis management?

- Children and adolescents respond well to exercises and bracing due to growth flexibility.
- Older adults may require slower, low-impact exercise and focus on bone health and balance.
- Management is individualized based on bone density, mobility, and overall health.

30. What is the most important factor for long-term spinal health?

Consistency in **posture awareness, spinal exercises, strength and flexibility training, nutrition, and lifestyle habits** is the key to preventing progression, reducing pain, and maintaining function throughout life.

Conclusion

Kyphosis, whether mild or severe, is more than just a postural concern—it is a reflection of overall spinal health, muscular balance, and body mechanics. While it can develop from age-related changes, poor posture, congenital factors, injuries, or medical conditions, it does not have to dictate the quality of one's life. With early recognition, consistent management, and a proactive approach to spine care, individuals can maintain mobility, reduce discomfort, and prevent progression.

Understanding that the spine is not an isolated structure but a dynamic pillar connected to every movement, organ system, and even emotional state is key. Good spinal health supports better breathing, circulation, digestion, and nervous system function, making it central to overall well-being. Therefore, addressing kyphosis is not simply about improving appearance—it is about enhancing daily function, energy levels, and long-term vitality.

In many cases, a combination of targeted exercises, posture training, lifestyle adjustments, and when necessary, medical intervention, can dramatically improve outcomes. For older adults, maintaining bone density through proper nutrition and weight-bearing activities is crucial. For younger individuals, cultivating healthy posture habits early can prevent future spinal deformities. For those already experiencing advanced kyphosis, modern treatment options—from physical therapy to surgical correction—offer hope for better alignment and comfort.

The journey to a healthy spine is not a one-time fix but a lifelong commitment. Simple habits such as regular stretching, mindful sitting, ergonomic workspace setups, and avoiding prolonged slouching can make a significant difference over time. Just as one invests in cardiovascular health through diet and exercise, spinal health demands the same dedication.

Ultimately, kyphosis serves as both a challenge and a reminder—our bodies are adaptable, but they require care. By taking responsibility for spinal wellness, staying active, and seeking help when needed, it is possible to live not only free from the limitations of kyphosis but with a stronger, more resilient back. In doing so, we protect not just the structure of our spine but the freedom, independence, and quality of life that a healthy spine makes possible.

THE END

Printed in Dunstable, United Kingdom